Andreas Ganz
Bernhard Johannes Schmidt

AF199036

Plaintext compact

Early Childhood Autism

Understanding = Helping

Andreas Ganz
Bernhard J. Schmidt

Plaintext compact
Early Childhood Autism
Understanding = Helping

© 2019 Bernhard J. Schmidt,
Oberwarmensteinach, Germany
All Rights reserved.

ISBN: 978-3750419049

translated from
Klartext kompakt.
Frühkindlicher Autismus
Verstehen = Helfen
© 2016 Bernhard J. Schmidt,
ISBN: 978-3741293719

Production and Publishing:
BoD – Books on Demand, Norderstedt, Germany

Bibliographic information of the German National Library:
The German National Library lists this publication
in the German National Bibliography; detailed bibliographic
Data are available online at http://dnb.dnb.de.

Dedicated to all those who,
in the spirit of dr. Ignaz Semmelweis,
wrestling for truth in their work.

Table of content

I. PREFACE

After the books on autism in general and the Asperger syndrome in particular, it is now still to treat the field of early childhood autism.

All previous books serve as a basis and are largely valid for people with early childhood autism - but must be expanded in their application and understanding accordingly. And again, this is about a compact presentation of the knowledge necessary for the understanding of early childhood autism.

From this knowledge alone already results in the possibility of and ability to help and support.

In the field of autism, the developmental dynamic approach we have outlined is new, but not so in the support of people with intellectual disabilities.

This is all the more surprising, at least at first sight, because autism is defined as a "profound DEVELOPMENT DISORDER".

Experts for whom the view presented here is too short, are referred to corresponding textbooks with the reference to apply the already established developmental dynamics in combination with the already outlined sociopsychological view also on autistic people.

II. INTRODUCTION

If a child receives the diagnosis of "early childhood autism," this means turning away from the idea of any developmental potential and turning to a static "judgment." Parents and relatives are deprived of any hope of a significant improvement in the autistic child's problems and largely normal development through the diagnosis and underlying misconceptions sold as certainties. Psychiatrists, psychologists and "professionals" are given a static view with the advice derived from giving the autistic children the best possible care home [see e.g. Poustka et al. (2009)].

The view represented here by us is the exact opposite! Every child goes through a development, each child has the chance - with appropriate support - to expand his boundaries, to shape his life. Although to varying degrees depending on the degree of disability.

However, early childhood autism as a "profound DEVELOPMENT disorder" offers many easy ways to support the child - if one understands the autistic child and his or her particular perception. The development-dynamic approach outlined here has been used intuitively by some support programs for decades (see Chapter V: Practice).

Now these intuitive applications are supported by a corresponding theoretical foundation.

*„Each stage of development provides a chance to create experiences for children that will help them master earlier stages that may have not been mastered the first time around. **It's never too late.**"*
[Greenspan, Stanley I.; Wieder, Serena (2006)]

1 How is this positive view possible?

The question should really be more, why this positive view has been hidden in early childhood autism so far? Because in the area of children with intellectual disabilities, this has long existed. If one replaces the words "intellectual disability" with "early childhood autism" in the following quotation (without equating them!), Then we are in the development dynamic perspective:

„It has been shown that timely support for different developmental aspects can improve their global functioning (Greenspan & Wieder, 1998, Guralnick, 1997). The findings of Spitz (1946), Mahler et al. (1975) and Bowlby (1951) on the social and emotional development of children also apply to disabled children. A child with an intellectual disability is first and foremost a child who, despite his limitations, has opportunities for

11

development. This optimistic perspective has today replaced the old conceptions of an immutable state. Menolascino (1977) and Wolfensberger (1972) assume that development is a lifelong process for all people, including mentally handicapped people, with individual intensity, speed and severity, of course. "
[Dosen, A. (2010), translation by B.J.S.]

Dosen even cites as reference the already cited authors Greenspan & Wieder, but does not take the step to apply its and also its own developmental dynamic approach to early childhood autism.

Years ago, Lingg & Theunissen (2000) had a developmentally dynamic approach for children with intellectual disabilities, but not for autistic individuals.

Both at Dosen (2010) and Lingg & Theunissen (2000), the change of perspectives within the respective book is massive. Across all forms of potential mental disability, a dynamic approach to development is advocated.

However, all of this is suddenly forgotten when changing to the presentation of autism.

But why do science and research deny autistic children the possibility of a (positive) development?

Why is early childhood autism still represented as static and immutable to this day?

Why is it that parents and relatives are deprived of hope,

and that support and help for autistic children is virtually suppressed?

2   The three mistakes of autism research

The refusal of a development-dynamic view and thus also the development of corresponding support programs for autistic children, are based on three fundamental errors of autism research.

2.1   The "refrigerator mother" trauma

A first development-dynamic approach led into a scientific as well as a human catastrophe. Searching for possible causes of autism Leo Kanner already suggested that a lack of maternal warmth and affection can be a cause. This assumption was continued by Bruno Bettelheim in 1967 in his book "*The Empty Fortress*". Due to a massive shortening and lack of discussion or review of the approach of Bettelheim, the "refrigerator mother" was subsequently identified as the cause of autism.
And with devastating consequences, especially for the mothers of autistic children.

More about this topic can be found in Schmidt, Bernhard J. (2019) "*The Refrigerator Mother Myth. A Rehabilitation of Bruno Bettelheim.*"

This first development-dynamic approach was mainly related to the emergence of autism and led to wrong conclusions with at the same time both for the parents and for the autism research traumatic consequences. Because further investigations showed that autism is to a large extent genetically conditioned and thus the mothers are not to blame for the development of autism.

2.2   Static instead of dynamic development

As a result, the "autistic child was spilled with the bath". The field of developmental dynamics has been considered mined in the entire autism research, nobody seemed to once again burn their fingers on the sensitive topic.
And with dramatic consequences:
„*For sixty years, treatments for ASD have focused on the symptoms of the condition, rather than on the underlying problems. As a result, goals for individual children have often been limited to changes in behavior, and the long-term prognosis for many children with the disorder has been deeply pessimistic. **Prevailing assumptions about***

***the nature of autism have limited the kind of progress
and future expected for these children.*** "
[Greenspan, Stanley I.; Wieder, Serena (2006)]

Although it has been described how negative
environmental interaction in children with intellectual
disabilities can lead to mental disorders, this is not
extended to autism.

*„On the one hand, we recognize that mentally
handicapped people are capable of getting mentally ill
regardless of their mental disability. On the other hand,
we understand that certain circumstances of the life
situation of many mentally disabled persons significantly
increase the risk of disease. Conditions that contribute to
a higher incidence of mental disorders in people with
mental disabilities compared to the general population
are, in addition to an environment that is generally less
in need of care - especially in large institutions - often a
pronounced self-esteem problem, impaired contact and
communication skills, limited or inadequate Possibilities
of articulation and assertion of one's own desires as well
as at the same time understatement and overburdening
that repeatedly lead to experiences of frustration and
make one's own, narrowly set boundaries painfully
palpable.
Compared to these great psychosocial burdens are only*

15

limited possibilities for self-help and usually only a small amount of social support. "
[Lingg; Theunissen (2000), translation by B.J.S.]

Again, it is enough to replace the words "mental retardation" with "infantile autism" in order to address the problems as well as opportunities for the development of autistic children and adults.

In the developmental dynamic model for children with intellectual disabilities, Anton Dosen describes four areas that influence the development of the child. They are the

1.) biological dimension
2.) social dimension
3.) functional dimension
4.) developmental dimension

„*For example, a baby born with a brain disease may be limp, remarkably calm, lacking in vitality and "good" (biological dimension).*
Because it is so quiet, it can receive little attention of the environment and thus less stimulation for its development (social dimension). Such a child develops more slowly, whereby all mentioned functions can remain underdeveloped (functional dimension). As a result of the

delayed development, the child can not sufficiently participate in the environmental dynamics, which may result in limited interactions. This in turn does not adequately stimulate biological conditions (development dimension). Changing one dimension (for example, social interactions as parents change their interactions through information and education) there are changes in the other three dimensions. " [Dosen, Anton (2010), translation by B.J.S.]

As soon as one applies a developmental dynamic perspective to autism, the difference between "early childhood" autism and "late-childhood" (!) Asperger's autism becomes immediately obvious, as we will see in Chapter III.4.
And also the possibilities to support and help autistic children becomes clear.

2.3   Semmelweis reflex

After the "fridge mother" disaster and the resulting static view, which has denied autistic children a positive developmental possibility as far as possible, the autism research commits just the third big mistake that will cause damage to autistic people and their parents.
Neither do autism researchers show willingness to

perceive and review a development-dynamic and socio-psychological theory - nor are they prepared to deal with corresponding support programs. [Schmidt, B. J. (2016/2) „Autismus. Wenn Händewaschen hilft.“]

„Semmelweis's reflex describes the notion that the scientific establishment rejects a new discovery without sufficient scrutiny and fights rather than supports the author.

... The conceptualization was coined by the American author Robert Anton Wilson and named after the Hungarian doctor Ignaz Semmelweis. Semmelweis attributed varying levels of childbed fever to poor hygiene among doctors and hospital staff, and sought to introduce sanitary codes. ...

During his lifetime, his findings were not recognized and rejected by colleagues as "speculative mischief".“
[Source: wikipedia.de, translation by B.J.S.]

Just as the majority of Ignaz Semmelweis's colleagues refused to wash their hands, and as a result many women died in childbirth at that time, today autism research is refusing to switch to a development-dynamic perspective. A comprehensive, effective and adapted support of autistic children becomes a stroke of luck.

Because as a result of a false, because static perspective of autism research, parent organizations such as "autism

Germany" (including the therapy centers operated by them) are blind to development-dynamic, strength-oriented and child-centered support programs such as Mifne (Israel), Son-Rise® (USA), Floortime / DIR® (USA) and AuJA (Germany).

The primary goal should be to publicize and develop these approaches. To make these support programs both better known and to provide them with a previously missing theoretical basis are the main concerns of this book.

3   Summary

At the beginning of this chapter was the question of how the positive view expressed here regarding early childhood autism is possible.

The answer to that is now easy.

It's the simple correction of the three mistakes of previous autism research through two small steps.

The first step is towards social psychology, as outlined in Schmidt (2015/1). So the step towards understanding that autism is not a "disruption of social interaction and communication", but a "lack of unconscious group communication".

The second step is the extension of the developmental dynamic point perspective, which is available for children with intellectual disabilities, to autism. So the return - despite "fridge mother" traumas - to developmental psychology. As will be seen in the following with several quotes, it often only requires the exchange of the words "mental disability" against "early childhood autism" to understand that the supposedly static "profound developmental disorder" is a possible (!) but not necessary disruption of development. And also to understand where the difference lies between "early childhood" and "late childhood" autism. And as a result, how autistic children can be helped, how they can be understood and supported in their own way.

As long as this paradigm shift is not carried out by the science and parent organizations, on the one hand valid research results are not possible and on the other parents and their autistic children will suffer from a lack of (static) understanding and refusal of adequate support.

III. AUTISM

Since the new social-psychological autism theory has already been described in detail in Schmidt, BJ (2015/1) and Schmidt, BJ (2015/2), we limit ourselves here to a brief summary of the most important aspects that are necessary for understanding the following development-dynamic perspective.

1   Autism is not a disease

Autism is to be distinguished as a genetically caused special form of sensory perception as well as social interaction of acquired autistic behaviors (see also Chapter IV.1 Autism and Disability). Through this special perception and interaction, which is briefly described below, autistic individuals have above all an increased vulnerability depending on the respective socio-cultural environment. In appropriate environments, however, autism can be beneficial to the survival of the group and thus an ESS (evolutionary stable strategy).
How the interplay of environment and interaction can affect the development of autistic individuals will be discussed below.

2   Hypersensitivity / stimulus filter weakness

Autism is often accompanied by a decreased sensibility in the perception of the inner world, e.g. from hunger, pain ... but above all a greatly increased sensory sensitivity when seeing, hearing, smelling and feeling. Disturbing stimuli, such as the ticking of a clock, other people's conversations, etc., can not be automatically faded out due to irritation filter weakness.

What can be an advantage in a natural environment, for example as a hunter, quickly leads to a sensory overload in a stimulus-flooded affluent society. Taking into account and registering these sensory features is a central basis for all support programs.

„Children show us their own solutions to their sensory processing system challenges. It's up to us to recognize the solution and figure out a way to expand on it by making it interactive."

[Greenspan, Stanley I.; Wieder, Serena (2006)]

3   Social Psychological Perspective

Autism is not, as very often misrepresented especially by "self-advocates", simply a hypersensitivity in combination with a stimulus filter weakness, ADHD, anxiety disorders, dissociative personality structures ...

The central point for understanding autism is the lack of unconscious group communication.

It has long been known in autism research that autistic people lack facial expressions and gestures, that the voice of autistic people is often very monotonous and not very modulated. It is also known that autistic people hardly mirror or imitate their counterparts and do not speak small talk. Social psychology has shown for decades that exactly these points, ie facial expressions, gestures, imitation, reflection, as well as small talk, serve the unconscious group communication and the "social grooming".

Autism is not a "disturbance of social communication and interaction", but the absence of unconscious group communication.

And with consequences not only for communication and interaction, but also for orientation in the world.

„Children who can't read and respond to social signals—facial expressions, gestures, body posture—have a hard time knowing what to do and when to do it. Long before

children can speak, caregivers let them know what is dangerous and what is safe by a look, a sound, or a tone of voice or by pointing.“
[Greenspan, Stanley I.; Wieder, Serena (2006)]

3.1.a   Unconscious group communication as "autopilot"

The unconscious group communication serves as an "autopilot". NT people (neurotypical people - as opposed to autistic people) are unconsciously oriented towards the group. In a natural environment or highly regulated and ritualized society (such as in Japan), this is not particularly noticeable. In a socio-cultural environment that has been characterized in recent decades by the dissolution of existing structures in almost all areas, the ability to unconsciously orientate oneself towards the group is of particular importance.

Autistic and even autistic children, due to a lack of orientation in the group, the environment often appears as incomprehensible and unmanageable.

[see also Schmidt, B.J .; Ganz, A. (2016)]

Also in the following quote is again "mental disability" by "early childhood autism" to replace.

„Does a person with intellectual disability have an environment that is "unbearable" for him, that does not create meaning, which for example is constantly over- or under-challenged, regulated, suppressed and in no way corresponds to his developmental potential, strengths, talents, needs and interests he form "symptoms".
These are expressions of a "self-healing attempt", that is, the conspicuous behavior is fed by a self-regulatory persistence against the negative influences.
The behavioral disorders or mental disorders therefore have a positive meaning and demonstrate in this case a usefulness for the maintenance of the personal system.
At the same time, it becomes apparent that it makes no sense to want to change the behavior of the individual.“
[Lingg; Theunissen (2000), translation by B.J.S.]

INTERaction and COMMUNicaton always take place in a socio-cultural environment, and must always be considered socio-psychologically, especially when disruptions occur.

3.1.b   Communication and Interaction

Communication and interaction are basically one and the same. Communication is always interaction and vice versa. Meaningful can be distinguished:

- verbal interaction

- nonverbal interaction

and

- conscious interaction

- unconscious interaction

Due to the culturally overemphasized verbal interaction, which is often restricted in autistic people, and the overlooking of unconscious interaction, misunderstandings and disturbances inevitably occur.

All humans, including autistic people, are social (!) beings and need a successful interaction with the environment to develop them - right from day one.

Interaction is always shaped by (unconscious) expectations, which are mainly caused by the socio-cultural environment. For example, in contrast to our culture, Japanese people have the expectation of the interaction partner that he does not look them in the eye, shows no feelings (through facial expressions and gestures) and does not shake hands.

Therefore, if autistic individuals encounter an (unconscious) expectation of unconscious group communication that autistic individuals can not fulfill, disruption of the interaction will have to occur.

Autistic people are often excluded from social (!) interaction because of the lack of unconscious group interaction. But this is, as already stated, of crucial importance for a positive personality development.

3.1.c   Gender Differences

The ratio of diagnosed autistic individuals is about 4 male to 1 female autistic. So far, due to the static and isolated view of this phenomenon was unexplainable and led to bizarre theories such as the 'extreme male brain' - "theory" by S. Baron-Cohen.

But with all legitimate equal rights - men and women, boys and girls behave differently in terms of communication and interaction. And society also meets the genders with different expectations.

As usually the "males" compete with each other for the "females", female humans, that is also autistic women, are confronted with much more interaction offers than boys / men.

Also, the hurdles to be overcome are different.

From the perspective of interaction as a necessary condition (which we shall discuss in the next chapter) for a successful development, the differences in both the frequency of occurrence and the development itself of autistic men and women become understandable.

Further remarks on this area can be found in Schmidt, Döhler, Döhler (2018) "*Autism - Sexuality - Relationships*".

4   Development Dynamic Perspective

All children develop through different stages. For decades, this has been studied by developmental psychology and there are several developmental models for explanation. So far for children with and without mental disabilities, but not for autistic children.

„The first scientific publications on the developmental approach to the phenomenon of intellectual disability date back to the 1940s (Piaget & Inhelder, 1947, Werner & Strauss, 1939). Later, this topic was further elaborated

*by Zigler (1961, 1971), Cicchetti (1984), Burack (1990), Hodapp et al. (1990), Greenspan (1997a) and many other authors. The basic premise here is **that people with an intellectual disability do not fundamentally differ in their psychosocial development from other people, but the development process takes longer and eventually ends up at a lower level than with non-disabled people.*"
[Dosen (2010), translation by B.J.S.]

Again with this quote, you just have to swap the words "mental disability" for "early childhood autism". Again, although Stanley I. Greenspan is called by A. Dosen, it nevertheless denies autistic children a dynamic developmental perspective.

However, unlike children with mental retardation, development in autistic children does not have to be delayed or at a lower level.

Decisive is the understanding of the peculiarities of perception, communication and interaction of autistic people as well as comprehensive support.

„For these reasons, ASD should be viewed as dynamic, not static. A static trait is fixed—the child will be this way no matter what the environment context, or

circumstances. A child's blue eyes are unlikely to change over time or due to changing circumstances; eye color is a relatively fixed trait. Dynamic traits, on the other hand —associated with many factors, including feelings and emotions—are changeable. The three core abilities identified above are dynamic processes: they can and do change—more for some children than for others, and more with certain kinds of treatment programs than with others. Professionals disagree as to the degree to which these abilities can be favorably influenced, both in general and in any particular child. Our view is that these abilities can change significantly and that a prognosis can be determined by only one factor—the child's actual progress. Many factors—including home environment, treatment program, an maturation of the child's nervous system—influence his or her progress. ***The only reliable indicator is the child's learning curve over time. The steeper the slope, the better.*** "
[Greenspan, Stanley I.; Wieder, Serena (2006)]

Without going into various theories of developmental psychology comprehensively, there are four areas that make up the development of a person, whether autistic or NT-human. What applies to the development of NT people, that also applies to people with intellectual disabilities - and also applies to autistic people!

4.1   Four strands of development

Both the interaction with the environment and the development of a human being starts in the womb. And a person's development, though different in intensity and flexibility at different times, is never quite complete. This also applies to autistic people.

„*It could be shown that by timely support of different developmental aspects, an improvement of the global functional level of these people can be achieved (Greenspan & Wieder, 1998, Guralnick, 1997). The findings of Spitz (1946), Mahler et al. (1975) and Bowlby (1951) on the social and emotional development of children also apply to disabled children. A child with an intellectual disability is first and foremost a child who, despite his limitations, has opportunities for development.* **This optimistic perspective has today replaced the old conceptions of an immutable state. Menolascino (1977) and Wolfensberger (1972) assume that development is a lifelong process in all people, including mentally handicapped people, with individual intensity, speed and severity, of course.**"*
[Dosen (2010), translation by B.J.S.]

Although Greenspan & Wieder is mentioned again, there is no development-dynamic perspective in the chapter on autism. Again, autism is considered purely static and isolated. So it is not surprising that the "DIR / Floortime" approach (see chapter Practice) by Greenspan & Wieder for the early support of autistic children is not mentioned. Not in the case of A. Dosen, not in Lingg & Theunissen, in autism research and in "autismus Deutschland".

„It is best to view ASD in a dynamic framework that considers all the factors that influence the child's development over time.
We advocate considering ASD (including Asperger's Syndrome) not as a fixed disorder that you either have or don't have, but as a dynamic process in which certain biological or neurological challenges affect development. *The degree of progress possible depends on the amount of neurological impairment, but rather than assuming a fixed disorder, practitioners should try to move each child through the stages of emotional and intellectual development to the best of the child's ability.“*
[Greenspan, Stanley I.; Wieder, Serena (2006)]

With the help of the socio-psychological perspective, the dynamics of development or its disturbance in autistic people becomes even clearer than in Greenspan & Wieder.

The four strands of development are:
      1.) Neurobiological and physical maturation
      2.) Development of homeostasis
      3.) Development of the cognitive basis
      4.) Socio-emotional development
These all start at the same time, but take different lengths. And all four strands need a successful interaction with the environment for successful development.

Sensitive phases of development

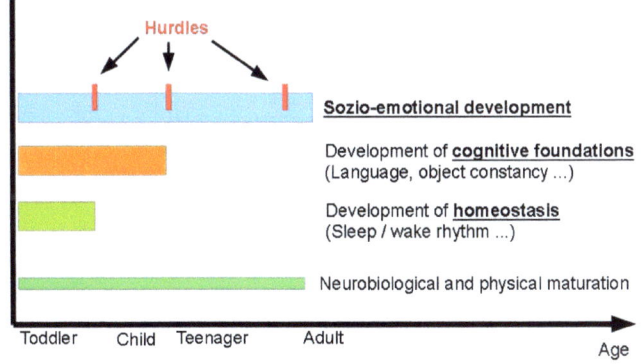

© 2016 Bernhard J. Schmidt

It is already clear from the graph that depending on the time of occurrence of a disruption of the interaction different development strands are affected, and thus the effects can be very different.

4.1.a   Neurobiological and physical maturation

The basis of all other developmental strands is the neurobiological and physical maturation. Only by creating the necessary neurological and biological prerequisites will the child be able to learn, for example, grasping, walking, talking .... Often, several strands of development are required at the same time, such as acquisition of language. Children of deaf-mute parents who communicate using sign language have been found to have speech prior to the physical maturation of the speech tools.

Just because a child does not speak does not mean it has no language (developed)!

4.1.b   Homeostasis

At the beginning of the development is mainly the development of homeostasis, so the physical balance. These include the very areas that autistic children often have problems with, such as the regulation of digestion, sensory integration and the sleep-wake cycle.

The development of homeostasis is also dependent on the interaction with the environment.

Without the unconscious orientation and imitation of other people's behaviors, autistic people are already struggling and need a good external structure - even more so than children with intellectual disabilities.

„*Treatment of sleep disorders*
Educational strategies
The focus is on providing comprehensive information to the environment about the basic physiological needs of the child. Parents need to know that for children with an intellectual disability, achieving physiological homeostasis during the early stages of adaptation may be much more difficult than with a non-disabled child. They need to learn how to help the child achieve a normal sleep-wake cycle. They should necessarily seek professional advice.

A stable regularity of activity and inactivity of the child as well as the structuring of the environmental conditions in relation to the spatial arrangement as well as on the sensory input are important.

If the environment itself is barely able to provide the necessary structure to the child because of internal and external problems (for example, psychological problems of the parents, unfavorable social environment), the

35

entire milieu must be included in the treatment. "
[Dosen (2010), translation by B.J.S.]

The development of homeostasis is usually completed in the transition from toddler to child.

4.1.c   Cognition

Even though people can learn and develop themselves intellectually throughout their lives, the basics of this must be created in childhood.
These are mainly learned through interaction with the environment and in the beginning in the form of games.

If there is a disruption of the interaction, it also leads to a disruption of the development of cognitive basics!

Starting with the formation of (sensory) perception and sensory integration in all areas to the complex acquisition of language.

„Disruption of speech development with average action IQ often leads to problems in the overall psychosocial development of the child with social anxiety, maladaptive behavior, autism-like behaviors and depression.
In non-intellectually disabled children under 3 years with

a delayed speech development, Irwin et al. (2002) show that these children also lagged behind in their emotional development and showed more behavioral problems (withdrawal, depression, less social contact) than non-speech-delayed children. This has been explained by the fact that the lesser expressive means of expression make these children less able to regulate and socialize their behavior and express their desires, needs and emotions. Problems of language development always have a negative influence on school learning and the contact with other children. "

[Dosen (2010), translation by B.J.S.]

On the one hand, the development of the cognitive foundations in turn has a strong influence on the socio-emotional development. On the other hand, however, it must always be remembered that the interaction underlying the development or its disruption is massively shaped by the expectations of the interactive environment! We will discuss this in detail in a later chapter.

In the central points, the development of the cognitive foundations in the transition from child to adolescent is completed.

4.1.d   Socio-emotional development

The culturally conditioned one-sided focus on cognitive development alone has largely overlooked the importance of socio-emotional development. As a result, for example, dissociative personality structures in autistic individuals (with normal cognitive and at the same time incomplete socio-emotional development) were falsely equated with autism [see also Schmidt, B. J .; Ganz, A. (2016)].

„Deep developmental dysfunctions
In the foreground of the scientific study of these disorders are the biological, sensory and cognitive aspects.
The emotional development of these people has so far received little attention.
However, day-to-day care practice has shown that people are difficult to understand in their basic emotional needs and social behavior because of their particular emotional developmental processes. ***This can lead to interaction problems with behavioral problems and mental disorders.*** " [Dosen (2010), translation by B.J.S.]

The socio-emotional development also lasts the longest and there are three hurdles in the way that must be overcome.

These are the transitions from

> 1.) Toddler (with the mother as the primary caregiver) to the child (with the family and their immediate environment as an interaction environment);
> 2.) child to adolescent, with the outgrowth of the family and the new orientation to peers;
> 3.) adolescents become adults, with the expansion of the interaction environment from the peers to the "world".

If these transitions are already difficult for NT people with "autopilot", that is unconscious orientation on the group, then these hurdles are understandably more problematic for autistic people.
For autistic boys, however, they are much more difficult than for autistic girls due to other gender interaction patterns and role expectations [see also: Schmidt, Döhler, Döhler (2018) "Autism – Sexuality - Relationships"].

4.2   Three influencing factors

All strands of development are influenced by three factors:

1.) by age,
2.) the socio-cultural environment and
3.) the interaction.

4.2.a   Age

Although it may seem trivial, it is important to point out, especially in autism, that development is a dynamic process. And so that a "developmental disorder" is always a disruption of development and thus the disruption of a dynamic process. And this dynamic process called 'development' takes place on a time axis where 'age' describes a point on the time axis.
Although the development can sometimes be faster and sometimes slower (called developmental delay) - but ultimately it follows automatically a continuous sequence of largely constructive steps. So a conscious and targeted gripping can take place only when the skeleton and the muscles are designed accordingly.
In the process of development, there are always

"sensitive phases" that offer a window of opportunity to develop certain skills.

„*Sensitive phases are defined as those periods of rapid growth of certain regions of the brain in which sensitivity to sensory stimuli is particularly pronounced, which differentiates and specializes these areas for their specific functions. For example, the sensory phase for the development of vision is in the first 6 months after birth. When an inborn cataract is surgically corrected in a child within the first 6 months, there are no adverse effects on vision.*

However, if the lens opacity persists for more than 6 months, vision is irreversibly damaged. Children with ongoing ear infections during the first two years of life may later experience significant hearing problems.

Children who have been barely involved in verbal communication in their early years are affected in their language development.

The appropriate external stimulation is therefore very important for the development of brain functions during certain periods of life (sensitive phases).

Even in the case of damage to certain brain regions (eg in the cerebral cortex), their function can be taken over by another area of the cerebral cortex. This ability is called the plasticity of the brain.

Thus, e.g. if the linguistic center is damaged in a child under the age of 3, the function of speaking is taken over by the other half of the brain. "
[Dosen (2010), translation by B.J.S.]

Sensitive phases are both possibilities for the quick acquisition of important skills, but at the same time, as the name implies, represent particularly vulnerable areas. **The successful interaction with the environment is always required to develop the skills, and disturbances of the interaction lead to massive problems.**

With advancing age, the development and training of skills slows down more and more - until it turns into the reversal, namely the increasing loss of skills.
However, this also means that as the development progresses, people become more and more "hardened" and thus less susceptible to disturbances of the interaction with the environment.

4.2.b   Socio-cultural environment

The second major area of influence on development lies in the socio-cultural environment. Development never takes place in a vacuum but necessarily requires interaction with the respective environment. As a result, humans are adapted in their development to their own environment - as long as it does not interfere with the interaction.

The socio-cultural environment spans from the general (in part gender) expectations, assumptions and demands of culture to the manifestation of the technical change in the environment, including the living conditions of the family in which the child's development takes place initially.

Depending on the particular culture, the expectations regarding the behavior of and the interaction with an individual can differ considerably.

And the gestures and facial expressions used for communication also have different meanings in different contexts. By early mimicking the behavior of the environment, NT people adapt automatically to the respective valid rules and behavior of one's own culture, one's own environment.

In addition, of course, the sensory environment is strongly influenced by the sometimes massive technical changes in the once-natural environment.

At the same time, the socio-cultural environment will affect the families. Affects the values, structures and expectations of family members. And also affects the sensory design of the apartment, for example.

All these points have a massive influence on the development of the individual.

It must be noted that the socio-cultural environment, at least for autistic people, has changed dramatically in the last few decades, which can at least partly explain the strong increase in autistic diagnoses.

On the one hand, neutral, side of a socio-cultural environment, for example, the Buddhist monastery with low sensory disturbances, structured daily routine, ritualized processes, little verbal communication ... we find on the other, for autistic negative, side of a flooded affluent society in the "default -Mode ", which is also characterized by the loss of solid structures and rituals.

4.2.c   Social Interaction

Development does not take place only in a vacuum (but in a socio-cultural environment), but always (!) requires social interaction. Attempts to grow children without social interaction, e.g. finding out the "original language" always ended with the death of the children. And "Hospitalism" shows impressively how much people are dependent on social interaction. This also applies to autistic people!

Autists can, want and have to participate in successful (!) social interaction!

And the "disruption of social interaction and communication" should not be viewed as static and isolated, but is always a dynamic process of interactions between the individuals involved in the interaction.

„For example, an "early disorder" often cited by mentally handicapped infants may result from their supposed passivity if they fail to attract the attention of their caregivers (e.g., lack of, reduced or altered vocalization, lack of motor activity).
In this case, basic interaction experiences are missing, which significantly affects both cognitive and affective development (lack of basic trust). A study by Papousek et al shows that children with two months react with unequivocal discomfort when mothers even for a moment, by closing their eyes, reduce their attention to childish expressions, look away or simply sit with their faces rigid, expressionless. First, the children try to face the mother's gaze in order to normalize and control the interactions. If this does not succeed, a typical protest behavior or a "depressed toned turn away" (Papousek 1989, 119) can be the result. "
[Lingg; Theunissen (2000), translation by B.J.S.]

Although autism is not caused by "refrigerator mothers," that does not mean that autistic people do not depend on a successful interaction for their development.
But on the contrary.

Autism as the absence of 'unconscious group communication' carries in it the high risk of disrupting 'social interaction' and thus the massive disruption of development as a dynamic process.

Thus, the support programs that we will present in the practical part are aimed primarily at building a positive interaction between mother / parents as primary caregivers and the autistic child, as well as the creation of a corresponding (sensory) environment.
By understanding the child's perspective and adapting to the communicative needs of the autistic child, astonishing positive developments are possible that have been erroneously denied to the autistic.

5   Autism as Vulnerability

Central to the understanding of autism is that it is not a "disorder" or "disease" but an increased vulnerability to the development of a disorder of interaction. And as a result, a disruption of development.

As an example of the difference between "disorder" and "vulnerability", people with red-blond hair and pale complexion should serve.

Depending on the intensity of UV radiation, these people are much more likely to get sunburned - and much more pronounced.

Belonging to the red-blond type is thus not a disease, even if significantly more often sunburns occur, but an increased vulnerability depending on the environment. In this case, depending on the UV radiation. This can, however, e.g. be increased by both socio-cultural processes (ozone hole) as well as the geographical location.

Problems (sunburn) thus arise from the vulnerability and inter alia the interaction with the socio-cultural environment.

IV. EARLY CHILDHOOD AUTISM

From the point of view of developmental dynamics, it immediately becomes more than clear where the difference between "early childhood autism" and "late childhood" autism, also called, for example, Asperger syndrome, lies.

Depending on the age or stage of development, in which a "disturbance of interaction" occurs, different areas of development are affected.

If the disorder occurs at an early stage where the basic developmental steps are not yet complete (hardened), the consequences resulting from the disruption of the interaction can be far more serious. It is therefore understandable why problems with, for example, the sleep-wake cycle as part of the homeostasis still to be developed are frequently to be observed in early childhood autism. It also becomes clear why problems can arise in the development of language and other cognitive abilities.

However, the later a disturbance of the interaction occurs, for example, in Asperger syndrome, the less developmental strands are still sensitive and can be negatively affected. The most problematic area is then the socio-emotional development.

The frequently observed discrepancy between normal cognitive and at the same time lagging socio-emotional development in Asperger's becomes understandable [see also: Schmidt, B. J .; Ganz, A. (2016)].

Sensitive phases of development

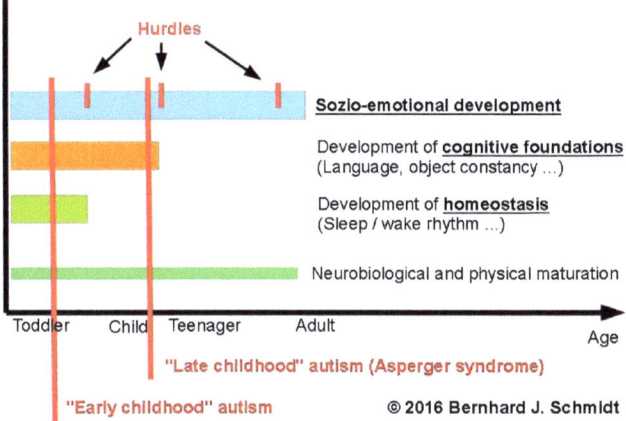

However, a disruption of interaction is and always will be a dynamic process between those involved in the interaction and the environment. That you can respond to a disturbance, no matter when it occurs, and eliminate it! Thereby the further way of a positive development is released again.

The elimination of the interaction disorder presupposes both the understanding of autistic perception and behavior as well as the adoption of the perspective of the child, as we will present in the practical part on the basis of 'child-centered' approaches.

1   Autism and disability

There is a strong relationship between autism and disability. On the one hand, congenital autism and the resulting disruption of interaction can lead to the development of disabilities.
On the other hand, sensory or intellectual disabilities can lead to autism-like symptoms - that's well known.

„Autism-like behaviors of blind children are probably primarily due to early attachment problems and therefore to be understood from a development perspective.
As a result, behavioral problems such as withdrawal, aggressive and autoaggressive behavior, separation anxiety and depressive states can arise.
In addition, problems are to be expected in the course of the first individuation phase (18 to 36 months of life), when children want to replace their caregivers with their uncertainties, fears and ambivalences. "
[Dosen (2010), translation by B.J.S.]

Intellectual as well as sensory disability can be innate as well as acquired.

However, it is always based on a 'disturbance of interaction'. On the one hand, for example, by a visual impairment, on the other by the lack of 'unconscious group communication' in autistic people.

As autistic behavior is therefore always (only) a symptom or the result of a disruption of the interaction!

All children, whether "normal" or disabled, can develop, albeit perhaps to varying degrees.
But they need understanding, and help and support based on it.

2   Goals of help

So far, due to the static and isolated view and the refusal of a developmental dynamic approach, the question of goals of help for autistic people has been insufficiently addressed.
If you deny autistic children a development from the beginning, then the question of goals also makes little sense or will be answered only superficially. As a rule, the goal of "therapeutic" intervention so far has been to adapt autistic people to social expectations and norms, such as looking in the eyes or giving a hand and reducing unwanted behavior.

But even autistic people have a right to mental health, to the development of their personality.

„From a psychodynamic and system theoretical perspective, mental health arises when the following conditions are met:
- a harmonious personality development,
- a private place in society,
- a self-responsible functioning,
- a positive future perspective. "
[Dosen (2010), translation by B.J.S.]

The current situation of autistic people in Germany, however, looks very different.

„Being marginalized and excluded from social participation and the primary labor market, autistic people have low health-related quality of life and an increased mortality risk.
Autistic individuals are particularly often victims of bullying and commit suicide more often than average."
[Schmidt, B. J. (2016/2), translation by B.J.S.]

Unfortunately, the cultural focus on the cognitive domain alone often overlooks the importance of socio-emotional development.

But for a "harmonic personality development" this also plays a central role in autistic people.

Although the mediation of cognitive content is given great attention, at the same time the emotional development is neglected. But:

„Emotion always comes before behavior. The child needs to enjoy relationships with parents, peers, and teachers in order to learn. So, rather than focusing on the behavior, we focus on the underlying emotional state. ***When the child finds pleasure in relating and learning, the behavior improves.*** *"*
[Greenspan, Stanley I.; Wieder, Serena (2006)]

More in the practical part.

3   Possibilities of help

Before we turn to the possibilities of help and support, briefly summarize the essential points needed to understand autism.

Autism from a socio-psychological perspective is essentially characterized by

   1.) the absence of unconscious group communication. It follows

- the lack of "autopilot" and thus difficulties with orientation

- often the exclusion of social interaction, exclusion of groups, bullying ...

- anxiety and stress

In addition come

2.) hypersensitivity and irritant filter weakness. From these follows

- Stress

- Risk of phobias, learned helplessness, ... [see also: Ganz, A .; Schmidt, B. (2016)]

- Retreat (from social interaction)

If one does not continue to deny autistics a developmental dynamic perspective, then it becomes clear that the development of autistic individuals, as described, depends on

    1. the socio-cultural environment and

    2. social interaction

Aids and support programs must therefore aim, at least initially (until "hardening"), to adapt as much as possible to the socio-cultural environment and social interaction to the sensory and communicative needs of autistic people. Only in this way will a healthy development of the autistic to the goal of a healthy personality become possible.

3.1   Socio-cultural environment

As already stated, development always takes place in a socio-cultural environment. This is, at best, neutral, as the example of the Buddhist monastery shows, but at worst very harmful. There is always a certain spread within a culture, depending on whether you live, for example, directly on a highway in the city or in a village. Depending on this, the three central spheres of influence of the socio-cultural environment will clearly differ on the development:

- the sensory loading or overloading,

- the orientation enabling social structures, as well

- the expectations of the behavior of others.

3.1.a   Expectations

People are always under the pressure of society's expectations and (unconsciously) orient themselves to them. Parents try at the same time, mostly unconsciously, to pass on these expectations to the children. This means that parents meet their children with the cultural expectations.

„Of course, not only the infant's behaviors or experiences can trigger misinterpretations, critical interactions, communication and developmental processes. Equally important for early disorders are specific attitudes, reactions, and communicative messages from caregivers that may be difficult to understand, ambiguous, irritating, or not "fit" for the child (Spitz, 1967). If, for example, there are overly high demands for performance in the face of a displacement or non-intentional disability as well as a strict standard of normality, there is a high risk that the children in question may feel overwhelmed and react with fears or feelings of rejection leading to neurotisation (Einkoten, compulsive behavior, inhibition of aggression, aggressive

breakthroughs, autoaggressive behavior) and can often lead to the blockage of sensorimotor and cognitive competence.

On the other hand, feelings of guilt and over-reliance can promote an under-demand or lack of risk-taking behavior of the child, dependencies and narcissistic-aggressive tendencies as well as complicate the ego-finding and autonomy process.

All in all, we can say that a disabled person suspected of having such early disturbances will have difficulty as adults in dealing with his social environment competently, and he becomes a problem for his caregivers because of his so-called 'behavioral disorders' and not just that because of the poorly developed ego function, but also because of the basic emotional experiences developed at this early stage of life such as mistrust, disappointment and anger.

Delayed cognitive development, poor maturation of psychic structures, adaptive learning processes, and a responsive and agile environment are inextricably linked together.

The result is a personality attributed to qualities such as anxiety, low frustration tolerance, impulsiveness, increased distractibility, unrealistic self-concept and the like - qualities that condense into classifiable diseases under unfavorable living conditions." (Gaedt 1987 b, 118f.)." [Lingg; Theunissen (2000), translation by B.J.S.]

The expectations of our culture are, among other things, the response of unconscious group communication (facial expressions, gestures, imitation ...) and behaviors such as hand giving, looking into the eyes and showing feelings. However, these are precisely the expectations that autistic children can not fulfill, which is why autistics are often falsely perceived as rude and repellent, and at the same time marginalized.

The basis for the understanding of the autistic child and thus for help and support is the removal of any (unconscious) expectations of the child.
Autistic people perceive the world differently and communicate differently - and therefore can not live up to cultural expectations.
The necessary approach to dealing with autistic children should be more akin to discovering a new continent.
Anyone expecting the same plants and animals when they discover a new continent as in their homeland, will be disappointed.
On the other hand, anyone who goes on an expedition with open eyes and no expectations will be rewarded with many new impressions.

That means: one should observe the (autistic) child without expectations and with open eyes - without judging.

„The Vital Role of Observation
We always begin an evaluation by simply observing the child; we conclude by coaching parents to bring out the best the child can do. Every child operates within a wide range of abilities. The key point is that the diagnosis has to be based on the top of the range. If the child can walk sometimes, the child can walk. She may fall sometimes, but she can walk. If the child can relate with others sometimes, he can relate, and we can help him to relate more. Understanding what the child can do at her or his very best is necessary to making the diagnosis.
Often, assessment conditions—noise in the room, a stranger the child has to deal with, various assessment tasks, and so forth—show the child only at the bottom of his range. That's important information: it helps an assessment team understand the child's individual differences and unique patterns.
Once a team has identified both the top and bottom of a child's range and observed the primary symptoms we have described here to be present even in a situation comfortable for the child, it may diagnose ASD. Or the team may notice that the child can relate, communicate,

and think creatively and abstractly, but not in a noisy environment. It may then assess the child for a regulatory disorder that leads him to lose his abilities under certain conditions of stress—a very different diagnosis than autism." [Greenspan, Stanley I.; Wieder, Serena (2006)]

Not without reason, however, subsidy programs are often used by parents, because the tensions between the

a) society's expectations of both parents and their autistic children,

b) needs of parents and

c) the non-judgmental treatment of one's own child, if possible without special expectations

are strong.

Raun K. Kaufman on his parents:
"*They persisted and persevered. Not knowing what the future held, not requiring my reciprocation of their love, care, smiles, and cheers, they gave me every chance.*" [Kaufman, Raun K. (2015)]

Unfortunately, disappointment with the personal needs and expectations of the parents is often accompanied by rejection by the environment and exclusion of the parents from social communication (with isolation as a consequence).

A persistence of the parents on the social expectations against (autistic) children will hardly be able to change this.

Expectation means that, for example, it is not a problem if a dog does not talk (which it usually does not), but if a child does not talk, it seems like a huge problem.

And of course you want - rightly - that your own child is talking. But not because of your own expectations, but because language is the door opener for the human world, and therefore important for THE CHILD!

The disappointment of (unconscious) expectations has in the past led to three far-reaching errors.

To the wrong assumptions that autistic

- can not communicate

- do not want to communicate

- do not need social interaction for development.

The opposite is true, however.

In addition, (unconscious) expectations lead to wrong assessments of autistic behavior. Instead, as the name ABA (applied behavior analysis) suggests, the behavior of autistic children is not analyzed for their meaning, but the behaviors that meet expectations are trained, and the unwanted ones are trained off.

In contrast, child-centered approaches, which we will introduce in the practice section, see autistic behavior as a meaningful adaptation of the child. Instead of the question "How can we train off unwanted behavior?" the question is asked, "Why does the child behave in this way, for which underlying needs is autistic behavior a symptom?"

The conscious letting go of (unconscious) expectations is thus a central requirement for the support of autistic children.

3.1.b   Sensory environment

Due to the progressive mechanization of our world, the sensory environment has changed dramatically in recent decades - to the detriment of all people with a hypersensitive perception.

The traffic has multiplied just as much as the general noise - light and air pollution have increased ...

And also in the domestic area, technology and wealth have left their mark. There, too, the degree of sensory stimuli has risen massively.

It is therefore not surprising that the programs presented

in the practical part always have the creation of a low-stimulus environment as a prerequisite.

„Discovering the Child's Sensory and Motor Profile
To help children be comfortable in the world, clinicians
and caregivers must first learn by careful observation
which sensations help children become calm and
regulated, which ones overwhelm them, and which don't
pull them in enough. Whatever the infant or child's age,
you the caregiver need to observe how she responds to
different types of touch on different parts of her body.
Experiment with different Sounds—high- and low-pitched
noises, the normal human voice—and different degrees of
volume to see which ones draw the child's attention
more. Do this with each of the senses. This helps you
determine which senses to emphasize as you draw the
child into your world.“
[Greenspan, Stanley I.; Wieder, Serena (2006)]

The observation and consideration (and, if necessary, modification) of the sensory environment as well as the reactions of the child are therefore of particular importance.

And not only in the direct interaction, but also with regard to the child's reaction to external stimuli.

A stimulus-flooded environment causes stress in the child - and stress stands in the way of learning and therefore also development [see also Schmidt, B. J .; Ganz, A. (2016)].

Apart from the detachment of (unconscious) expectations, the adaptation of the environment to the sensory peculiarities of the autistic child is the second central starting point for help.

3.1.c   Orientation

Development does not happen in a vacuum. Children need a successful orientation towards the environment for their development. This orientation occurs in two ways:

1. on external structures such as e.g. regular eating or sleeping times,
2. through unconscious group interaction, imitation and synchronization.

Due to the lack of unconscious group interaction, imitation and synchronization, autistic people rely solely on orientation to external structures.

If these too are largely lacking, orientation and thus positive development are difficult.

And without orientation, the world appears as incomprehensible, as chaotic and threatening.

„Does a person with intellectual disability have an environment that is "unbearable" for him, that does not create meaning, which for example is constantly over- or under-challenged, regulated, suppressed and in no way corresponds to his developmental potential, strengths, talents, needs and interests he form "symptoms".
These are expressions of a "self-healing attempt", that is, the conspicuous behavior is fed by a self-regulatory persistence against the negative influences.
The behavioral disorders or mental disorders therefore have a positive meaning and demonstrate in this case a usefulness for the maintenance of the personal system.
At the same time, it becomes apparent that it makes no sense to want to change the behavior of the individual. "
[Lingg; Theunissen (2000), translation by B.J.S.]

Many, at first glance, strange and undesirable behaviors of autistic individuals are actually an attempt to navigate a world that appears chaotic and hostile.

Rituals and stereotypes create within the person an order that is not perceived in the world. The aim of a support is therefore always the mediation of the world as structured and friendly through social interaction. This presupposes the willingness to engage with the perception of the autistic, to accept the supposedly strange behaviors as meaningful and to meet him first in his world. Because in this own world of stereotypes and rituals, the autistic child feels safe and secure, has the feeling of control and manageability.

This should go hand in hand with the creation of external, clear structures in which the autistic child can orient itself.

Only if the child can perceive the world around him as structured and thus understandable, it will want to leave its own world of safer structures and rituals and find the necessary orientation for development.

3.2   Social interaction

To understand autism and autistics, the distinction between "unconscious group" and "social" interaction is central.

Although autistic individuals lack the unconscious group interaction and can not participate in it, so often (unconscious) expectations, for example, of parents are disappointed.

Nevertheless, autistic people are capable of social interaction and need it for their development.

Due to the lack of unconscious group communication,

however, autistics are often excluded from social communication or do not take place.

The interaction partners that are important for the development of the various strands change.

In the beginning, the interaction between the (autistic) child and the mother takes center stage.

This interaction then expands to the family, then to peers and the "world" in the form of other adults, work colleagues ...

Since the "early" childhood autism, the disturbance of the interaction, as already shown, occurs at an early stage, the consideration of the mother / parent as the interaction partner of the child is necessarily the focus.

3.2.a   Interaction mother/parents - child

The mother / parents are in the area of early childhood Autism crucial!

Not only is it their interaction with the child that is necessary for its development, they also (or not) provide the structure in which the child can orient.

And above all, they are the first to recognize the child's problems and then turn to an unfortunately long search for help, support or diagnosis.

But the sooner the child and his behavior are understood and positive support begins, the better. The sooner the disturbance of the interaction is removed, the better the autistic child will be able to develop. Especially in the initial phase of development, in which on the one hand all strands are still sensitive, but the child is also extremely vulnerable, every week counts.

„The positive effect of early intervention is also related to the emotional and social changes in the family. Through the structured and targeted approach, the parents can be strengthened in their positive expectations and attitude towards the child and thus in their social interactions. This undoubtedly promotes the child's social and emotional development. Overall, there are significant improvements in motor and language, emotional stability of the child and social behavior, as well as improvements in the mother-child relationship and overall family situation.“ [Dosen (2010), translation by B.J.S.]

What A. Dosen correctly represents, takes into account the 'family first' approach of Greenspan & Wieder, which we will discuss in more detail in the practical part. 'Family first' means the beginning of early intervention BEFORE the diagnosis! Because until this is asked, usually takes a lot of time, too much time.

The most important points for the autistic child are

1. the trust of the mother / parents in his ability to develop,
2. the knowledge that also autistic children want to communicate and interact, and need it for their development,
3. as well as the willingness to say goodbye to your (culturally conditioned) expectations.

V. PRACTICE: CHILD-INITIATED COMMUNICATION

Although the social-psychological and development-dynamic approach we have developed in autism is new, support programs have been developed for decades that not only fit in well with our approach, but are above all suitable for supporting children with early childhood autism.

As well known ABA, TEACCH and PECS are, so unfortunately unknown are the following briefly, without claim to completeness, presented approaches. This is probably due to the previously false, because isolated and not socio-psychological / developmental dynamic "understanding" of autism.

It is time to pay more attention to these support programs and to develop them further.

Even though each support program is slightly different, the common foundation of the four approaches

1. AuJA - Accept autism and act, Döhler / GERMANY
2. Floortime/DIR® , Greenspan / USA
3. Mifne ('Turning Point' in Hebrew) / ISRAEL
4. Son-Rise-Program®, Kaufman / USA

is the "child initiated communication".

"The children show us the way in, and then we show them the way out."
[Kaufman, Raun K. (2015)]

In all of the above approaches, the autistic child is in the foreground, the behavior of the child considered as meaningful from the perspective of the child and at the same time as an interaction attempt - and not as otherwise evaluated as negative. All approaches are also based on a development-dynamic perspective.

The central points of three approaches - Floortime / DIR®, Son-Rise® and AuJA - are presented below. This presentation of the most important points, of course, can not be a complete representation of all aspects of the respective funding program and does not replace their own study programs.

The book by Raun K. Kaufman (2015) "Autism breakthrough", which is coherent as well as readable, offers on an intuitive basis deep insights into the phenomenon of autism as well as the practical handling of autistic children.

But let's first turn to the "Floortime / DIR®" approach of Greenspan & Wieder.

1 Floortime/DIR®

Parts of the theoretical foundations of the Floortime / DIR® program are already familiar to you from the previous quotations from the book by Greenspan & Wieder (2006).

Based on these theoretical foundations, the "The Floortime Center®" 2004, which was led by Stanley Greenspan's son, among others, emerged. In this the "DIR / Floortime®" program for families is offered. Still necessary and at the same time illuminating the peculiarity of this approach is the explanation of the abbreviation "DIR":

„In the name "developmental, individual-difference, relationship-based approach,"developmental" refers to the six stages or levels [...], "individual-difference" refers to the unique way a child processes information, and "relationship-based" refers to our understanding of the learning relationships that enable a child to progress in his development. The DIR model builds on the three insights articulated above to create intervention programs based on which of the six developmental levels a child has reached, on her individual processing profile, and on the interactive relationships that best support her

development. The DIR method of analysis thus enables
parents, educators, and clinicians to make assessments
and plan treatment programs tailored to individual
children with ASD. "
[Greenspan, Stanley I.; Wieder, Serena (2006)]

On the one hand, Floortime / DIR® is a development-
dynamic approach that analyzes the individual
differences of the children and makes them the basis of
further support.
Emphasis is placed on the emotional relationship with the
child and not on cognitive development. Because the
(positive) emotion is the basis for learning. It is always
the child and its development in the center - and not the
expectations of parents or society.

„The most basic difference between the major
approaches is in their goals. Developmental approaches
such as DIR/Floortime strive to help children build
healthy foundations for relating, communicating, and
thinking. In contrast, behavioral approaches (the most
intensive of which is ABA-Discrete Trial, developed by
Ivar Lovaas) work on changing surface behaviors with
structured tasks. In the most recent study of behavioral
approaches—the only one to use a true clinical trial
design (randomly assigning children to different

interventions)—Tristram Smith (a colleague of Lovaas) showed that these approaches produced only modest gains in educational areas and little to no gains in emotional and social areas, compared to control groups. And even in terms of the structured educational gains, only 13 percent of the children studied achieved the high-level educational outcomes that were claimed for much higher percentage in earlier studies (see Smith, Groen, and Wynn, 2000, in References). Also, a review in 2004 of all studies on ABA approaches by Victoria Shea showed that the original claims for their effectiveness have not been replicated (Shea, 2004, in References). Behavioral approaches, when successful, may change specific behaviors, but because they rely on repetition and highly structured learning, most children who learn tasks with this approach may perform the tasks only in the way they practice them. Therefore, they may not develop fundamental cognitive, language, or social capacities. contrast, what are broadly termed "developmental relationship approaches" tend to use naturalistic learning—that is, learning through interaction and discovery. The results are improvements in social interactions—engaging in imaginative play, forming friendships, getting comfortable with dependency and warmth, and the like—as well as advances in thinking abilities. This is not surprising, because these

approaches tend to work with foundation skills such as engaging, relating with others, and reading social signals, and to practice these in spontaneous learning interactions."
[Greenspan, Stanley I.; Wieder, Serena (2006)]

The goal is to help the child with special needs to go up the six levels of his or her development.

These are after Greenspan & Wieder:

1.) shared attention and regulation
(starts at 0 - 3 months)
2.) commitment and relationship building
(starts at 2 - 5 months)
3.) Targeted emotional interaction
(starts at 4 - 10 months)
4.) Long chains of mutual emotional signaling and joint problem solving (starts at 10 - 18 months)
5.) Creating ideas (starts at 18 - 30 months)
6.) Building bridges between ideas: logical thinking
(starts at 30 - 42 months)

"Floortime" means that the mother / parents ... go to the level of the child, that is, the ground and perform with the child the most important form of interaction for this development point - play! And that according to the supposedly funny rules of the child!

By engaging in the child's play, not only interaction, but also trust and an emotional attachment are established. Greenspan & Wieder does not overlook the fact that the first few months are crucial for the development of the child - unfortunately a diagnosis often takes too long. That's why they have developed the "Family First" approach.

1.1   Family first

The result of a major recent survey in England [Crane, L. et al. (2016)] among parents of autistic children has shown that, on the one hand, parents wait on average for about a year before they go to a specialist after first concerns about the development of the child.

The period up to the diagnosis and thus starting support lay on a further average of three and a half years! Both the time to diagnosis and the associated stress and subsequent support were often perceived as unsatisfactory.

From a developmental perspective, however, it immediately becomes clear that promoting the autistic child as early as possible is desirable and necessary. This is where "Family first" comes in:

„A Family First approach enables parents to help the child to learn to relate, communicate, and think while waiting for a professional screening, comprehensive evaluation, and the start of educational and therapeutic programs, and also after such programs are under way. Even if a screening does not identify ASD or other problems, this approach can only strengthen healthy development. If a child does show developmental delays and an evaluation suggests the need for a comprehensive treatment program, these initial steps parents carry out on their own can be refined and expanded with the help of an intervention team. "
[Greenspan, Stanley I.; Wieder, Serena (2006)]

ALL children need social interaction for their development - whether autistic or not.
And a successful interaction with the environment can only be of use - never hurt.

The family is therefore the most important starting point to enable or promote the development of the autistic child. The sooner the parenting training starts, the better. In doing so, the parents do not become such as at ABA, considered as a therapist, but as an interaction partner for their autistic children. The central point is therefore to make the parents understand the special interaction behavior of their children and to show them how they can communicate with their child.

„As we have discussed, the children with ASD and other special needs who make the most developmental progress are those who are engaged during most of their waking hours in healthy learning interactions tailored to their unique developmental needs. That's why families must be at the center of any intervention program. The Family First concept is supported by mounting evidence that, as discussed in Part I, certain formative child-caregiver interactions are essential for healthy social, emotional, and intellectual development and that these same practices can prevent or lessen the degree of developmental delay and can facilitate progress in infants and young children at risk for or already showing difficulties, including ASD."
[Greenspan, Stanley I.; Wieder, Serena (2006)]

The family is the central place for the support of autistic children - even before a diagnosis.

1.2   Floortime as a family concept

The family is the linchpin for all the advances of the (autistic) child. Development does not take place in a vacuum or at all, as hitherto mistakenly assumed in the field of autism, but always in a socio-cultural environment. And the family with all its members is at the beginning and thus with early childhood autism in the foreground.

"*Rather than talking about a child with special needs, we should talk about families with special needs, because when a child has uneven development—whether the cause is ASD or a severe language, motor, or other problem—the entire family has a challenge. Families have two primary ways of responding to a diagnosis of autism or other developmental problem. The positive response is to take the crisis as a cue to organize everyone in the family and the community to rise to the occasion, to find new ways of coming together and new constructive solutions. Certainly, many families and communities do just that in a crisis.*"
[Greenspan, Stanley I.; Wieder, Serena (2006)]

But the challenges for a family with a child with special needs are high. And the success of a positive approach to the situation is not self-evident.

„*Unfortunately, a different response all too often gets in the way of instructive one. The stress of the situation can lead to a narrow focus and rigidity, just as children who have ASD or other special needs can be rigid as a way to cope, families sometimes react the same way. We see this in the larger world, too; a crisis can cause polarization, an "us versus them" mentality, in a community. Becoming rigid, anxious, polarized; focusing in on a few details; and limiting one's perspective is, of course, a common response to stress that goes back to early human ancestors."*

[Greenspan, Stanley I.; Wieder, Serena (2006)]

Not only autistic people are prone to rigidity and focus, but also people and families (systems) under stress in general. Therefore, an analysis of the family system according to Greenspan & Wieder is the necessary basis:

„To help the child through the [developmental] steps [...] and apply the Floortime methods [...], the first job of a family is to figure out the relative strengths and vulnerabilities of each caregiver."

[Greenspan, Stanley I.; Wieder, Serena (2006)]

The greater the existing difficulties within the family, the greater the need for specialist support.
And the family system includes both the parents of the autistic child and his siblings.

1.2.a   Parents

Children are oriented towards their parents, including autistic children. And if the parents are not feeling well, they themselves have big problems, the interaction will not be easier. Only if the parents are well and any problems are / were eliminated, can a successful social interaction take place.
Only if reliable structures are available, the autistic child can orientate itself.

„A child's progress with a DIR/Floortime program requires parents who are emotionally very available. If their emotions are drained by marital strife; by anger, disappointment, or depression; or by exhaustion from their workload, it's very hard for them to provide their child what he needs. The heart of Floortime is the warmth and nurturing that you're conveying to your child so he will want to play with you rather than retreat into his own world."
[Greenspan, Stanley I.; Wieder, Serena (2006)]

Supporting an autistic child needs to involve the parents, but not only:

1.2.b   Siblings

Siblings of autistic children are the most important "ally" of the parents - but also have their own legitimate (!) claims.

The sibling children want to communicate with their little siblings! And often even have better access.

However, they also need the attention of their parents, as appropriate to their age and stage of development, as well as the siblings with special needs.

If, for example, the (autistic) child screams on the arm of the sibling - then is taken away by the parents after a few seconds, then the sibling feels "guilty" - but it is not! Such misunderstandings should be avoided.

Also siblings are part of the family, take part in the social interaction. And siblings may well suffer from the special needs of the autistic child.

„*It's the parents' job to help the sibling feel included in a constructive, not a burdensome, way. As we mentioned, you don't want to make the sibling into another adult by giving him or her too many responsibilities, nor do you want exclusion.*"

[Greenspan, Stanley I.; Wieder, Serena (2006)]

Only when the family system works with all its members, and when all can come to their own right, feel well and develop, the autistic child can also develop.

1.2.c   Emotion befor behavior

Contrary to the overemphasis on cognitive development and behavioral changes of the autistic child, the DIR / Floortime® concept is used in the positive development of emotions.

„Emotion always comes before behavior. The child needs to enjoy relationships with parents, peers, and teachers in order to learn. So, rather than focusing on the behavior, we focus on the underlying emotional state. When the child finds pleasure in relating and learning, the behavior improves."
[Greenspan, Stanley I.; Wieder, Serena (2006)]

The development-dynamic approach developed by us, which basically states that all development needs social interaction to succeed, shows how useful this preference for emotion is.
Without positive emotion, social interaction will fail. It would be good for all areas of the support of autistic people to adopt this view. The dissociative personality

structure with normal cognitive and lacking socio-emotional development, which frequently occurs in "late childhood autism", impressively demonstrates the necessity of paying attention to emotions and socio-emotional development.

1.2.d   Guidance by the child

The main difference to ABA, TEACCH and similar support programs is that DIR / Floortime® is aimed at the autistic child and his needs. The behavior of the child is not considered to be disturbing but to be meaningful and helpful from the child's perspective.
The question is not how to change the child's behavior, but why it behaves in this way.

„Why do we follow the child's lead? After all, historically, educators have long held that adults can't just allow children to do what they want to do, because children are creatures of instinct who would never become socialized if we just followed their lead. But in Floortime, we take our cue from die child because a child's interests are the window to her emotional and intellectual life. Through observing the child's interests and natural desires, we get a picture of what she finds enjoyable, what motivates her. If a child is staring at a

fan, rubbing a spot on the floor over and over, or always walking on her toes, these might seem actions that we want to discourage. But something about the behavior is meaningful or pleasurable to the child. Therefore, we always start off by asking the question, "Why is my child doing that?" To say simply that it's because he has this or that disorder doesn't answer the question. The child may have a disorder or a set of problems, but he is not the disorder or set of problems. He is a human being with real feelings, real desires, and real wishes. If children can't express their desires or wishes, we have to deduce what they enjoy from what they are doing. So in Floortime we begin by following die child's lead and joining him in his own world."

[Greenspan, Stanley I.; Wieder, Serena (2006)]

And also in following the guidance of the child again (unconscious) expectations can stand in the way.

„One of the most important things is to meet the child at his current developmental level. Parents often are disappointed that their child isn't playing the way they think he should be. If that enters your mind, it's an indication that you are not following the child's lead enough. To help the child be more purposeful, we want to treat what he is doing as purposeful. Start out by helping

him to do what he wants to do, then try to expand on that with him.“

[Greenspan, Stanley I.; Wieder, Serena (2006)]

Once again, it is about saying goodbye to (unconscious) expectations and meeting the child in his own world.

1.2.e   Challenge

In addition to the "leadership by the child" is a central point of the playful construction of "obstacles" as a challenge. But how can a "leadership through the child" work in parallel with "challenge"?

Greenspan & Wieder understand by "guiding through the child" the observance and benefit of the interests of the child.

The "challenge", ie the playful construction of obstacles, then takes place in the area that interests the child.

„*Following the Child's Lead and Challenging the Child at the Same Time*

As we've explained, the DIR/Floortime approach is based on the idea that emotion is critical to the growth of the mind and brain. Following the child's lead means following his emotions. We ask, "What is of interest to this child? What gives him pleasure?" Whatever it is, the

child's interest is our clue, our window into what he's feeling. So we watch closely to tune into his emotional world. Once we figure out what he's interested in, we use that to draw him further up the developmental ladder ..."
[Greenspan, Stanley I.; Wieder, Serena (2006)]

So the child is not required to do things that the child does not want to do (for example, put dice in corresponding holes) - but if a child plays with a car, for example, it is covered by hand; or you stand in the door as an "obstacle", which is opened and closed again and again by the child.
Or when the child desires to leave the interaction or walks alone through the room, an arm circle is formed around it, which the child must overcome. This is how the interaction with the child should be created.

„We build on the child's interest to help him move up the ladder of shared attention, engagement, two-way communication, shared problem-solving, and creative and logical use of ideas. That requires not just following the child's lead but also challenging him. So, when we say, "Follow the child's lead," we don't mean simply copying or imitating the child. We mean taking the child's cue in order to build new interactions and experiences. Every interest of the child—even aimless wandering—

can be turned into an interaction and a challenge that helps him move up the developmental ladder."
[Greenspan, Stanley I.; Wieder, Serena (2006)]

In diesem Punkt unterscheidet sich DIR/Floortime®️ deutlich vom „Son-Rise Program®️".

2   Son-Rise-Program®️

The Son-Rise-Program®️ is much more intuitive and practical than DIR / Floortime®️ and was developed in the 1970s by the parents Kaufman for their autistic son Raun K.
The "Autism Treatment Center of America ™️", founded in 1983, is today headed by Raun K. Kaufman and offers the Son-Rise-Program®️.
The main difference to "DIR / Floortime®️" is, among other things, the lack of the "challenge" of the child. Also, the child's repetitive and solitary actions are not interrupted by the Son-Rise Program®️, but are considered helpful to the child.

„The Son-Rise Program Vs. Floortime - A Comparison: ... Floor Time describes itself as child-centered and indeed encourages parents to follow the lead of their child, discover the child's interest, elaborate and build on

whatever the child is interested in and assist the child in his/her play rather than trying to direct the play in a particular direction. However, the parent is also encouraged to do "whatever it takes" to make play interactive. So, if a child begins to move away from a game, the parent is instructed to pursue the child, "insist on a response" or "playfully obstruct" in order to keep the child in the game. If the parent asks a question which the child does not answer, the parent is instructed to persist with this question until an answer is provided. So, it seems that Floor Time is only child-centered for as long at it serves the adult.

The Son-Rise Program, however, remains child-centered regardless of what the child is doing. There are no conditions on the child's behavior in The Son-Rise Program. If a child turns away from interaction to engage in a solitary activity, then the facilitator follows the child and joins him/her in that activity. The facilitator joins the child by performing the activity in a solitary way, not by trying to turn the solitary play into interaction. The facilitator will wait for the child to indicate that he/she is again open to interaction before trying to engage the child. If the child makes eye contact, makes a sound, speaks or physically moves towards the facilitator, these cues will be responded to by encouraging interaction in a playful, animated and fun manner. If the child then pulls away again, the facilitator will again go back to solitary play until the child indicates his availability again. This technique reveals a fundamental difference between Floor Time and The Son-Rise Program. ...

The Son-Rise Program operates from the belief that children engage in these exclusive or repetitious activities for a reason, and that usually the activity is curative in some way. ...

Floor Time suggests that if a child is perseverating on an activity, then one should do whatever one can to create interaction, not heeding the child's cues (e.g. their turning away or saying "no"), but persisting in the pursuit. ... "

[source: http://www.autismtreatmentcenter.org/information/son-rise_and_floortime.php]

At the same time, the sensory environment is taken into account and the creation of a non-irritating, non-distracting environment is an important issue.
And also the negative influence of stress on the child, its development and health is taken seriously and seriously.
The importance of anxiety and stress for the understanding of autism, the behavior of autistic people

as well as the development of disorders in autistic people has already been discussed several times, e.g. in Schmidt, B.J. (2015/1 and 2015/2) as well as in Schmidt, B. J .; Ganz, A. (2016).

The central goal of the Son-Rise Program® is to empower the autistic child to successfully participate in social interaction with society.

Four steps are identified on the way to social interaction:

1.) Eye contact and non-verbal communication

2.) verbal communication

3.) Interactive attention span

4.) Flexibility

And with the Son-Rise Program® as well, the path to achieving those goals is to follow the child's needs - rather than conflicting with the child.

„... *to enable you to help your child grow and learn while going with instead of against your child, bonding more with your child instead of doing battle with him. This leads us to a most important, paradoxically logical idea: overcoming autism is not about getting your child to change his behaviors. Really.*"
[Kaufman, Raun K. (2015)]

So it is not surprising that Raun K. Kaufman considers a total reversal of perspective to be necessary.

2.1   Total reversal

"It's time for a total reversal. Instead of focusing on your child conforming to your world, you want to become a student of your child's world. Let your child be the teacher." [Kaufman, Raun K. (2015)]

In order to be able to help an autistic child, one must first (learn to) understand the child and his behavioral patterns. This requires a non-judgmental observation of the child's behavior.

"First, we want to change the question we ask ourselves when seeking to help our child. Instead of asking, "What do I need to do in order to change my child's behavior?" we want to ask, "What do I need to do in order to create a relationship with my child?" Once we ask this question, everything changes. Our whole approach shifts. You want to begin to focus on doing your very best to see through your child's eyes. I'm not asking you to be psychic here. I'm talking about imagining, with every single interaction you have with your child, what this might feel like for your child. When you stop your child from stimming, how might that feel for her? When you take him to a noisy park and he's covering his ears, how

do you think that is for him? When your child seems engrossed in tearing paper into tiny strips, what do you think that experience is like for her? When your child talks incessantly about windmills, what is it that he loves so much about them?"
[Kaufman, Raun K. (2015)]

The observation of the child thus forms the basis for all further steps. Without the observation and understanding of the behavior of the autistic child, successful support is not possible.

2.2 Ambassador

Even without the theoretical concept of autism as "absence of unconscious group interaction" and consequently problems with understanding and orientation towards the behavior of others, the Son-Rise Program® understands how autistic children may perceive the environment, as well as the interaction with this, as alien.

"*You want interacting with others to feel totally nonthreatening, fun, exciting, and satisfying for your child. In fact, you want to sell human interaction. I mean really sell it. If you went up to your child and said,*

"Dude, I've got the best deal to offer you! It's called being part of our world, and it's really awesome. You know what the best part is? When you join us in our world, you get to stop doing all the stuff you love, and start doing all the stuff you hate! Doesn't that sound fantastic?" Now, no child or adult on earth is going to take that deal. And yet, that's the deal we usually offer."
[Kaufman, Raun K. (2015)]

The image of the "ambassador" very well reflects the meaning that the behavior of the parents in relation to the environment has for the autistic child.
The child will consider the behavior of the parent or environment as representative of this world.

„*YOU ARE OUR WORLD'S AMBASSADOR*
Have you ever met someone from a foreign country? Have you ever noticed that you attribute the characteristics of that person to the country from which he hails? If the person is pushy you think. People from that country are pushy. If the person is loud you think. People from over there are loud. If the person is respectful, you think, That country has a very respectful culture. Every single second that you are with your child, you are for better or worse, our world's ambassador. You represent the world of human interaction. Everything that

you do tells your child what it's like to be a part of our world. If you force or push, that tells your child that our world is one where she will be coerced. If you disapprove, that tells her that our world is a disapproving world. If you give control, that tells her that the interactive world is one in which she can feel secure and have autonomy. If you are approving, that tells your child that our world is an approving one. You are asking your child to permanently join you in your world. For this reason, it is critical that you remain extremely aware of the messages you are sending about what that world is like." [Kaufman, Raun K. (2015)]

2.2.a   Stimming

Self-stimulating behavior (stimming) has an important function in autistic children. The perception as wrong and undesirable with the aim to train off this behavior is wrong.
For autistic children, this is an important way to calm down in a foreign and hostile world.
Without unconscious group orientation, the autistic child is in a situation comparable to a stay in a foreign country with strange customs and manners.

„The people don't speak our language. They have cultural traditions that seem unfathomable—yet we're expected to follow them. Even flushing the (strangely arranged) toilet can seem like an exercise in code breaking. Why can't everything just be understandable?! And why won't people get off my back and stop expecting me to obey rules I don't understand?! Often, in these situations, we become less social. We seek to wall ourselves in. And we seek familiarity and control. The same is true for many of us when we start a new job, move to a new area, or marry into a family that's very different from ours. This is exactly what your child does. In fact, your child is so brilliant and so creative that he has come up with a way to handle both challenges at once: the stim. How does the stim do that? First, it enables your child to focus intently on one thing so that he can most effectively tune out the sensory bombardment that he is experiencing every moment of every day. (Interestingly, this is the same reason why some people meditate.)" [Kaufman, Raun K. (2015)]

As explained in Schmidt (2015/2), repetitive behavior of autistic people can be explained by anxiety and stress. This is also what the Son-Rise Program® understands.

„...., by doing the same exact thing over and over in a way that he can control, your child is, in essence, creating an island of predictability in an ocean of randomness. So, you see, your child is actually addressing both neurological issues with one behavior! He is doing the best, smartest thing that he can possibly do to address what is going on for him. In reality, your child is not behaving abnormally. Your child is behaving extremely normally in the face of the abnormal situation that he is facing."
[Kaufman, Raun K. (2015)]

And it is the task of the parents to provide the autistic child in a friendly way as an "ambassador" with security and orientation. Then, automatically the stimming will be less, the child will turn more and more to social interaction.

2.3   Relax

And the importance of stress in the negative sense and relaxation in the positive is emphasized.

„FIGHT-OR-FLIGHT SURVIVAL MODE

There is a preponderance of evidence showing that the vast majority of children with autism are living in a near-perpetual fight-or-flight state. ...

When your body is in fight-or-flight, you are basically in immediate survival mode. These are some key biological processes of this state.

- *Adrenaline (epinephrine) courses through your veins.*

- *Your heart rate increases.*

- *Blood vessels constrict (to prevent excessive bleeding).*

- *Blood flows away from your vital organs and into your arms and legs (to ready you for running or fighting).*

- *Lymphocytes from your immune system race toward your skin (in readiness for you being cut or bitten).*

Also, of particular relevance to your child:

Major, more vital, areas of your immune system shut down—while other areas become hyperactive.

    1.   Your digestive system shuts down.

2. *Physiological repair gets put on hold.*
3. *The brain gears up for quick, immediate, reflexive decision-making—rather than tasks such as learning and social interaction.*

And, importantly, cortisol and corticotropin-releasing hormone levels skyrocket. Cortisol is the major long-acting stress hormone in your body. It is secreted by your adrenal glands. Corticotropin-releasing hormone (CRH) is a stress hormone released in the brain—but now found in other areas of the body in children with autism. ... "

[Kaufman, Raun K. (2015)]

Impressively, Raun K. Kaufman describes the massive negative effects of stress, if they are permanent!

„However, we are not designed to stew in this state indefinitely. Fight-or-flight survival mode works in a short burst. Fight-or-flight survival mode for hours or days begins to cause detrimental breakdowns in the human body. Take this physiological situation and apply it to our children, and what do you get? Let's have another look at the last five bullet points above. Think about what happens if major areas of your child's immune system shut down, and she already has a compromised immune system (or if a child with an

autoimmune disease keeps triggering immune system overreaction). Or if your child's digestive system shuts down, and she already has digestive issues. Or if you are administering biomedical interventions designed to help your child's digestive, immune, and other systems rebuild —and major physiological repair is on hold in her body. Now also imagine trying to help your child to learn and interact socially when her brain is in this fight-or-flight state. Learning and social interaction are exceedingly difficult for our children when they are in this mode. Attention span is affected interfering with learning, and the child is in a highly self protective state, shutting down her ability to interact socially." [Kaufman, Raun K. (2015)]

Anxiety and stress thus have a massive negative impact on the autistic child, on his health and his ability to learn as well as to interact [see also Schmidt, B. J .; Ganz, A. (2016)]. Without a consistent reduction in anxiety and stress - not just in the child - all efforts to support the autistic child will go nowhere.

2.4   Trust

To reduce anxiety and stress and to be in contact with the child, building trust is a central issue. Only when the child trusts the mother / parent will the child want to engage in social interaction.

To build that trust, engaging in the child's behavior (rather than criticizing it) is of immense importance. And in the knowledge that the behavior of the child is not meaningless, but has an important and meaningful function for him.

2.4.a   Joining

Joining as the foundation of the Son-Rise Program® is the opposite of impelling desired behavior. But it is not simply the imitation of the child's behavior. Admittedly, the adult does the same thing as the child when he joins, but for himself, as well as the child. Only when the child, by itself, shows interest in interaction through, for example, a look, this interaction is begun.

„*Joining*
And this is where a true understanding of joining (and of autism) has real impact. Joining isn't a trick we use to sneak our child into a different activity or behavior. Joining is the way we enable our child to form a bond with us. We find that children become more interested in us, look at us more, and ism far less when we join. But these children do these things by choice—at their own

101

initiation. After our children bond with us, trust us. .uid feel safe with us—which they show us by initiating interaction—then we can challenge them to do and learn new things, ..." [Kaufman, Raun K. (2015)]

2.5   Confirm and celebrate

Part of a successful social interaction and the basis for a successful development of a child is the confirmation of his existence as well as his actions.

Due to a perception of the autistic child as "different" and his behavior as "unwanted", usually a confirmation is omitted.

The Son-Rise Program®, on the other hand, consciously focuses on celebrating the child and confirming positive behavior. Thus the autistic child experiences herself as desired, and at the same time the environment as friendly. In contrast, put yourself in the position of a child who is only rejected and scolded for his "unwanted" behavior ...

2.6   Control

Again and again, Raun K. Kaufman points out that while spontaneous or "normal" reactions of parents are understandable, they are counterproductive in autistic children. So the natural impulse will be to gain control of

the child, be it through control struggles.
But what seems intuitively correct leads to the opposite in autistic children, for whom the world seems incomprehensible and uncontrollable.
It is the abandonment of control that is of crucial importance to autistic children.

„*How Giving Control Generates Breakthroughs*
You love your child and value your child's progress.
That's wonderful and important. And I know that
sometimes it's easy to get single-mindedly caught up in
achieving a particular milestone with your child. In your
pursuit of your child's progress, though, it is essential to
temporarily relinquish any goal as soon as it causes a
control battle with your child. In fact, control battles are
one of the most disabling dealings you can have with
your child. You want to avoid them whenever possible
(except when safety is involved, of course)."
[Kaufman, Raun K. (2015)]

Only when the autistic child perceives the environment as understandable, friendly and controllable will it be able to open up to a social interaction.
This can not be done through control struggles, but only by giving control to the autistic child (as long as the behavior carries no risks).

The aim of the Son-Rise Program® is to train the weak "muscles" instead of "fitting in" them.

TEACCH and PECS are seen as crutches at best, but can also stand in the way of language development, for example.

The aim of the Son-Rise Program® is, as already stated, to enable the child to interact as far as possible with the environment. And for that, acquiring, for example, language, if possible, is of fundamental importance.

3   AuJA-Program

As the third and final, the only one to date in the German-speaking world, and still very young "child-centered" support program will be discussed.

As a parent of their autistic child, the Döhler family has been looking for ways to help their son.

From their own experiences with the Son-Rise Program® as well as the improvisational theater, the "AuJA - Autism Accept and Act" program was created in 2012. This is largely based on the Son-Rise Program®, but is also enriched by the elements of improvisational theater. The central place is the "space" in which the parents and volunteers offer the autistic child the opportunity for social interaction in a non-irritating environment.

In addition, both the well-being of the parents and the

child is taken into account and the activity in the "game room" is adjusted accordingly.
And the child can withdraw at any time, is not forced to interact.

A further successful development of the program for the German-speaking countries would be desirable, but Döhlers experience so far no constructive-critical support by, for example, the association "autism Germany" or other autism associations.
And unfortunately not by science and research in the field of autism / curative education.
As the AuJA program is still in its infancy and developing rapidly, we refer you to the website www.auja.org for more information.
There you will also find videos of the AuJA program.
In addition, a comprehensive film documentation is currently in the making.

4   Summary

Even if the funding programs differ in individual points - the much larger difference lies between the previously known ones like ABA, TEACCH, PECS ... and the child-centered ones presented here.
The change in the understanding of autistic behavior

towards the idea that it is meaningful and helpful from the point of view of the child leads to a correspondingly sensitive approach to the child.

The goal is not to get rid of "unwanted" behaviors, but to build a fulfilling interaction, especially on a positive emotional basis. Because this in turn is rightly understood as a prerequisite for the development of even cognitive abilities.

5 Criticism

Precisely because attention and further development of the above-mentioned support programs is desirable, the weak points should also be addressed.

5.1 Lack of Social Psychological Perspective

While all have a developmentally dynamic approach, the social-psychological perspective of autism is lacking (except in AuJA) as a "lack of unconscious group interaction".

Without unconscious group communication, autistics are not identified as members of an in-group, not even an out-group, are often excluded and marginalized and victims of bullying.

Although it is recognized that autistic children have

problems with orientation and the resulting anxiety and stress, but not why this is so (absence of the "autopilot"). However valuable the practical findings for the promotion of autistic children are nevertheless, so much does the theoretical foundation suffer from the lack of social-psychological perspective.
But this can be corrected in the future.

5.2 Socio-cultural environment

It is also overlooked that development always takes place in a socio-cultural environment that influences, among other things, the expectations of the parents, but also the sensory environment. But the expectations of society, teachers, employers, etc. are not fixed, but dependent on the socio-cultural environment and subject to constant change. All this affects the development of the autistic child.
It is therefore overlooked that the interaction partners are not limited to parents and family, but change greatly with the progress of development.

5.3 Changing interaction partners

If in the beginning the interaction with mother and family is in the foreground, this changes with the change from child to teenager.

The peers and the attempt of interaction with and orientation to these then emerges.

It is overlooked that relations, interactions always depend on all interaction partners.

„Peer Relationships
Children diagnosed with Asperger's Syndrome who are sufficiently verbal and academically skillful to be in a regular class but cannot get along appropriately with other children feel isolated and alienated. They can become very sad and depressed. They are aware enough to want to have friends and to be part of a social group, but they are also keenly aware of their lack of acceptance by Others. Teenagers and adults with similar developmental disabilities may experience the same feelings. "
[Greenspan, Stanley I.; Wieder, Serena (2006)]

The socio-psychological perspective shows the importance of exclusion and traumatization by the environment [see Schmidt, B. J.; Ganz, A. (2019/6)], which are based on fundamental (unconscious) group-dynamic processes and not on the autistic.

With the transition to the adult, the "world" as an

interaction partner stands opposite. Again, it is the socio-cultural environment that causes problems such as exclusion from the primary labor market.

So, even if older Asperger autists are seen as potential clients, and support programs are seen as suitable for them, both the diversity and reciprocity of interaction are overlooked.

„The best help for autistic people without mental disabilities would be a society in which they need no help!"
[Schmidt, B. J. (2015/2)]

5.4   Strong commercialization

Except for the AuJA program, which is run as a charitable UG and represents an emancipatory claim, all other support programs "suffer" from some massive commercialization.
This automatically raises the question of whether the well-being of the child (alone) is in the foreground.
Instead of providing necessary information to as many parents of autistic children as possible and empowering parents to support their children, too often the emphasis is on commercial success.

5.5   „Healing"

Along with the strong commercialization then goes in part the promise of a "cure of autism". This puts these support programs unfortunately in the vicinity of dubious methods such as MMS etc.

„I recovered completely from my autism without any trace of my former condition."
[Kaufman, Raun K. (2015)]

But it is precisely through the socio-psychological perspective of autism as a "lack of unconscious group interaction" that it becomes clear that there can be no cure in this sense. Much can be compensated, much achieved - but an autistic remains an autist, remains in the "task mode", and the "default mode" with unconscious group orientation, etc. remains a mystery.
And it's always the environment that reacts to exclusion, rejection and bullying to people who do not reciprocate unconscious group communication that can not be identified as "in-group".

5.6 As a supplement to the English edition

The following further criticisms are taken from Schmidt, B.J. (2019/5):

5.6.a Limits and dangers of child-initiated support programs

As good and appropriate as the child-centered support programs are for the "flight-type", that is, for autistic children who refuse contact with the world and have withdrawn completely into their own world, these programs also have their limitations and dangers.

5.6.b Limits

The playroom in which support program usually takes place is always an artificial world. And the interaction, as good as it is to re-establish communication in the beginning, remains artificial. So, these support programs are good for getting started with interacting with people. But social interaction is learned through social interaction - and that takes place in the real world with all its dangers and risks, and especially in peer groups.
Once the first stages of interaction within the playroom

have been achieved, further interventions such as social skills training would be necessary as offers.

And with the "fight" type, which explores the environment strongly, it does not make much sense to bring these children back into a playroom. Here, the opportunity should be seized to use exploration to build a relationship.

Likewise, the child-initiated support programs quickly reach their limits in aggressive behavior. Too much effort is made to build up an interaction so that, for fear of a renewed withdrawal of the child, there are hardly any limits to aggressive action.

5.6.c   Dangers

The biggest danger of child-initiated support programs is not to see the limits listed above.

For example, a family with a very aggressive juvenile autistic who had years of "playroom" was advised to use even more Son-rise® to solve the problem. Its own boundaries were ignored and instead followed the principle of "more of the same".

On the other hand, in almost all, not only the child-initiated support and therapy programs but also e.g. at ABA, made the parents "co-therapists". From now on, the behavior of the children will be documented by the parents from a "therapeutic meta-level", analyzed and, if in doubt, discussed with the children ("What does it matter to you if you throw the salt shaker?"). A normal interaction between parents and children, in which there is room for conflict and the child is once even reprimanded, is thereby prevented. But the social interaction with the parents - and that at eye level - is of central importance to development. Even the parents of autistic children should and must remain parents - and not become "experts in their own right".

Another, partly also from financial interests bred error is that of the "much helps much". The support program then determines the entire life of the entire family and is run around the clock as possible. You rush from appointment to appointment, from therapy to therapy.

"We no longer have friends but only people around us who pay for their participation in the therapies. We do not have any time left to go through the many therapies," says a mother. But how is the young autistic son of this mother to learn what friends are and how to deal with them, if the parents themselves have no friends?

6   Links

AuJA - Autismus akzeptieren und handeln,
Döhler / DEUTSCHLAND
www.auja.org

Floortime/DIR®, Greenspan / USA
http://www.thefloortimecenter.com/

Mifne ('Wendepunkt' auf Hebräisch) / ISRAEL
http://mifne-autism.com

Son-Rise-Program®, Kaufman / USA
http://www.autismtreatmentcenter.org/

VI. A FEW WORDS ABOUT DIETS

The ideas of a "cure" through diets, mostly with a strong ideological coloring, often come from the USA. That may not be surprising, since the diet is basically very unhealthy there. Almost 95% of the food is made up of industrially produced products, ie with high levels of colorings and flavorings, flavor enhancers and preservatives.

However, because autistic children often have problems with digestion, dietary "cure" seems very tempting. But the idea of wanting to heal autism through diet is based on a confusion of cause and effect.

Because autistics often have gastrointestinal problems because of the high level of stress, among other things, this does not mean that gastrointestinal problems cause autism.

If there are problems with the digestive tract, a solution should be sought in the correct order.

In the first place, however, must always be a clarification by a specialist done that not other (serious) problems are the cause!

1   Healthy balanced diet

First of all, a balanced diet must be taken into account. The food should be freshly cooked and, if possible, without preservatives, artificial colors, flavors and flavor enhancers.

2   Regular diet

Also should be eaten at regular times. This is especially necessary in infancy to build homeostasis.

3   Reduction of stress

Of fundamental importance is the reduction of anxiety and stress. The effects that stress can have on the digestive system have already been described in the chapter on the Son-Rise Program®.
A person in a permanent state of stress can hardly have a healthy digestion.

4   Reduction of individual components

If digestive problems persist after performing the above and following a medical examination, a full diet should not be introduced immediately. Try out which substance, whether gluten, casein, lactose ... the child reacts negatively (allergic) at all.
This saves you and your child a lot of stress and many additional problems.

VII.   EPILOGUE

Autists are not "empty fortresses", as a book by Bruno Bettelheim about autism begins.
Autists are also not callous automata without a chance of development, which at best can be trained by conditioning rudimentary behaviors and / or disturbing behaviors.

Autists are humans, are individuals with their own CVs and development paths.

Autists, like all other people, need social interaction for their development, need understanding, acceptance and affirmation.

And autistic people, like all other people, have a right to a healthy personality development.

Although it has long been known that mothers are not at fault for developing autism, mothers / parents are the most important interaction partners who can significantly influence the development of their autistic child through appropriate interaction.
If this promotion does not happen, that's usually not up to

the parents! But to "pretend science", and lack of understanding or knowledge in the various support structures.

And: "It is never too late".
Even though individual areas of development "harden", are no longer quite as flexible, the ability of an (autistic) person to learn and develop only ends with death.

This book is the "capstone" of the book series, which presents the new social-psychological and development-dynamic perspective.

Started with
"*Autistic and society. An angry change of perspective. Volume 1: Understanding Autism*"
[Schmidt, B.J. (2015/1)]
with the presentation of the new social-psychological perspective, and
"*Autistic and society. An angry change of perspective. Volume 2: Support for Autistic?*"
[Schmidt, B.J. (2015/2)]
as a representation of the diathesis-stress-model, the "default-mode" / "task-mode" theory, as well as the support possibilities in the area "development of resources", up to

"Plaintext compact. The Asperger syndrome - not only for Psychotherapists. "
[Schmidt, B.J .; Ganz, A. (2016)]
with the first comprehensive theory on the development of psychic disorders in autistic patients using the diathesis stress model, as well as presentation of diagnosis and therapy.
With the presentation of the first comprehensive development dynamics theory on (early childhood) autism as vulnerability depending on social interaction and socio-cultural environment in this book, now closes the theoretical as well as practical circle.

That past autism research has not yielded valid results even after several decades to date [Waterhouse, Lynn et al. (2016)], becomes immediately apparent from the new perspective.
The previous consideration and exploration of autism as static, isolated and "disorder" equals the notion that the earth is a disc.
It's time for a paradigm shift!

BIBLIOGRAPHY

Crane, L., Chester, J. W., Goddard, L., Henry, L. &
Hill, E. L. (2016).
Experiences of autism diagnosis: A survey of over
1000 parents in the United Kingdom. Autism,
20(2), pp. 153-162. doi:
10.1177/1362361315573636

Došen, Anton; Hennicke, Klaus (2010):
Psychische Störungen, Verhaltensprobleme und
intellektuelle Behinderung. Ein integrativer Ansatz
für Kinder und Erwachsene. Göttingen, Bern,
Wien, Paris, Oxford, Prag, Toronto, Cambridge,
MA, Amsterdam, Kopenhagen, Stockholm:
Hogrefe.

Greenspan, Stanley I.; Wieder, Serena (2009):
Engaging autism. Using the floortime approach to
help children relate, communicate, and think. 1st
Da Capo Press pbk. ed. Philadelphia, Pa.: Da Capo
Lifelong Books.

Kaufman, Raun Kahlil (2015):

Autism breakthrough. The groundbreaking method that has helped families all over the world. First St. Martin's Griffin edition. New York: St. Martin's Griffin.
Lingg, Albert; Theunissen, Georg (2000):
Psychische Störungen und geistige Behinderung. Ein Lehrbuch und Kompendium für die Praxis. 4., völlig überarb. und aktualisierte Aufl. Freiburg im Breisgau: Lambertus.

Poustka, Fritz (2009):
Ratgeber autistische Störungen. Informationen für Betroffene, Eltern, Lehrer und Erzieher. 2., überarb. Aufl. Göttingen, Bern, Wien, Paris, Oxford, Prag, Toronto, Cambridge, MA, Amsterdam, Kopenhagen, Stockholm: Hogrefe (Ratgeber Kinder- und Jugendpsychotherapie, Bd. 5).

Schmidt, Bernhard J. (2015/1): Autistic and Society. An angry Change of Perspective. Vol. I: Understanding Autism. Norderstedt: Books on Demand.

Schmidt, Bernhard J. (2015/2): Autistic and Society. An angry Change of Perspective. Vol. II: Support for Autistic? Norderstedt: Books on Demand.

Schmidt, Bernhard J. (2016/1): Plaintext compact. The

Asperger Syndrome – Between Bullying and Inclusion.
Norderstedt: Books on Demand.

Schmidt, Bernhard J. (2016/2):
Autismus. Wenn Händewaschen hilft.
1. Auflage. Norderstedt: Books on Demand

Schmidt, Bernhard J. (2019/1): Autism and the
Refrigerator Mother Myth. A Rehabilitation of Bruno
Bettelheim. Norderstedt: Books on Demand.

Schmidt, Bernhard J. (2019/2): Plaintext compact. The
Asperger Syndrome – for Parents. Norderstedt: Books on
Demand.

Schmidt, Bernhard J. (2019/3): Plaintext compact. The
Asperger Syndrome – for Teachers. Norderstedt: Books
on Demand.

Schmidt, Bernhard J. (2019/4): Plaintext compact. The
Asperger Syndrome – for School Assistants. Norderstedt:
Books on Demand.

Schmidt, Bernhard J. (2019/5): Autism – Flight or Fight.
New Perspectives on Challenging Behaviors.
Norderstedt: Books on Demand.

Schmidt, Bernhard J.; Döhler, Christiane and Deniz (2018): Autism – Sexuality – Relationships. Norderstedt: Books on Demand.

Schmidt, Bernhard J.; Ganz, Andreas (2016): Plaintext compact: The Asperger Syndrome - not only for Psychotherapists. Norderstedt: Books on Demand.

Schmidt, Bernhard J.; Ganz, Andreas (2019/6): Plaintext compact. The Asperger Syndrome – for Physicians. Norderstedt: Books on Demand.

Waterhouse, Lynn; London, Eric; Gillberg, Christopher (2016): ASD Validity.
In: Rev J Autism Dev Disord. DOI: 10.1007/s40489-016-0085-x.